Bikini Line Waxing

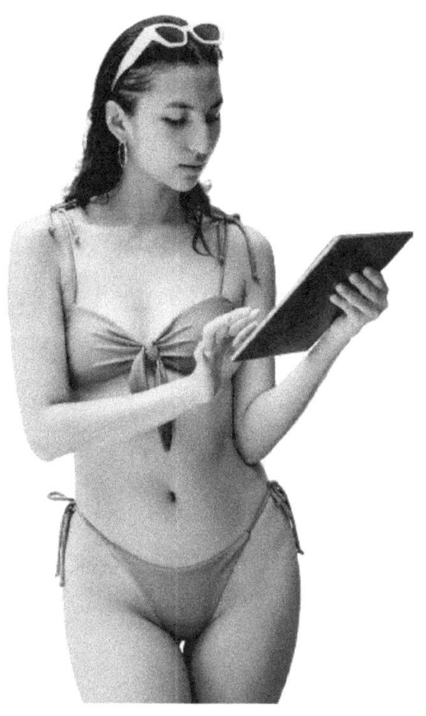

Homemade Organic DIY Hair Removal
Skin care

Carmen A Josephine

DISCLAIMER

Acknowledgment

I would like to express my heartfelt gratitude to all those who contributed to the creation of this book on at-home bikini line waxing for the summer. First and foremost, I extend my thanks to the readers, for your curiosity and interest in learning the art of hair removal. Your enthusiasm is what fuels the creation of such guides.

A special acknowledgment goes to the experts in the field of beauty and skincare whose insights and knowledge have formed the foundation of this book. Your expertise has been invaluable in shaping a comprehensive and informative guide.

I would also like to extend my appreciation to the entire team that worked tirelessly behind the scenes editors, designers, and researchers who played a crucial role in bringing this book to life.

Lastly, I am grateful to friends and family for their unwavering support and encouragement throughout this journey. It is your belief in me that keeps me striving to provide valuable content to those seeking to enhance their self-care practices.

With heartfelt appreciation.

Dedication

To all the beauty enthusiasts and seekers of confidence, this book is dedicated to you. Your desire to embrace self-care and enhance your natural radiance has inspired the creation of this guide.

To the individuals who believe that the journey to smooth, confident skin is worth every effort, this dedication is for you. May the pages of this book become a source of guidance, empowerment, and newfound knowledge as you embark on your hair removal adventure.

In honor of the countless moments you'll feel a surge of confidence, the sun-kissed days you'll cherish, and the self-assured smiles you'll proudly wear, I dedicate this book to your unwavering determination to look and feel your best.

May the insights shared within these pages become your compass, guiding you toward the ultimate goal: beautifully smooth skin and the undeniable confidence that accompanies it. Here's to you, your journey, and your undeniable beauty.

With admiration.

Table of Contents

Introduction

Welcome to the ultimate guide to achieving a flawlessly smooth and confident bikini line this summer! As the sun-kissed days beckon and beach escapades await, there's no better time to embark on a journey of self-care and grooming mastery. This comprehensive guide is your passport to mastering the art of bikini line waxing at the comfort of your own home.

Imagine the sensation of silky-smooth skin against the touch of your favorite swimsuit, the confidence radiating from within as you bask in the warm sunlight. Whether you're a waxing novice or a seasoned pro, this book is designed to be your trusted companion, leading you through each step of the process with expertise and precision.

Discover the secrets to a successful waxing session that goes beyond just hair removal. From selecting the right wax for your skin type to mastering the techniques that ensure minimal discomfort, we're here to demystify the process and empower you to embrace the summer season with open arms – and a radiant bikini line.

But it's not just about the waxing itself. We'll delve into the nuances of skin preparation, post-wax care, troubleshooting, and maintenance, ensuring that you not only achieve impeccable results but also enjoy lasting smoothness without the common pitfalls.

So, whether you're gearing up for that much-awaited beach vacation, a poolside soirée, or simply embracing the spirit of the season, let this guide be your ultimate companion on the journey to a perfectly groomed and confidently radiant bikini line. Your best summer starts right here – with the knowledge and expertise you'll gain within these pages.

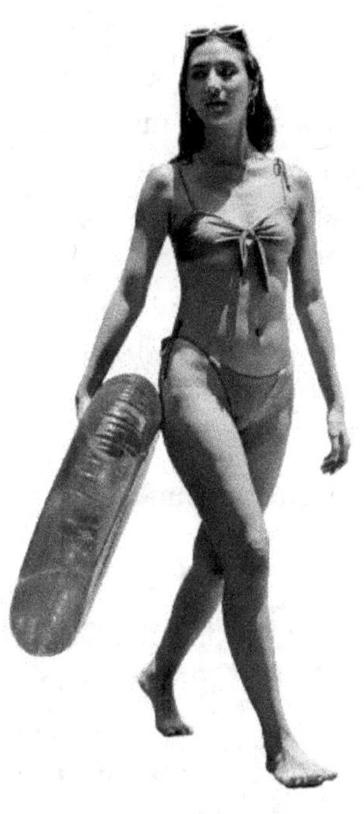

Chapter 1

Importance of Bikini Line Grooming

Grooming the bikini line has both a personal and a functional meaning; it is not only an aesthetic choice. In addition to cosmetic attractiveness, maintaining a well-groomed bikini line has the following advantages:

1. Boosted Confidence: A well-groomed bikini line can increase your self-confidence, helping you feel more relaxed and at ease in a variety of settings, including the beach, the pool, or just wearing your regular clothes.

2. Hygiene : The danger of infections and discomfort is lower when the bikini area is kept clean and free of sweat, debris, and bacteria.

3. Comfort: The chance of irritation from rubbing against garments and coarse hairs is decreased by grooming. Swimwear and tightly fitted clothing may feel more comfortable for someone with smooth skin.

4. Better Appearance: An attractive bikini line can improve the appearance of swimwear and lingerie, adding to a woman's polished and put-together image.

5. The Right to Wear What You Want: You can wear a variety of clothing styles with confidence and no concern about showing hair or discomfort if your bikini line is well-groomed.

6. Sensual and Intimate Self-Awareness: Grooming can improve sexual encounters by heightening your sense of sensuality and enhancing your self-assurance in close friendships.

7. Simpler Hair Removal: Regular grooming often results in finer regrowth, which makes subsequent waxing or shaving sessions less uncomfortable and more effective.

8. Summer-Ready: A well-groomed bikini line enables you to completely enjoy these experiences without feeling self-conscious, especially during the summer when beach trips and outdoor activities are popular.

In the end, how you choose to groom your bikini line will depend on your preferences. Feeling at ease, certain, and empowered in your own skin is the ultimate goal, regardless of whether you choose a clean shave, waxing, or any other procedure.

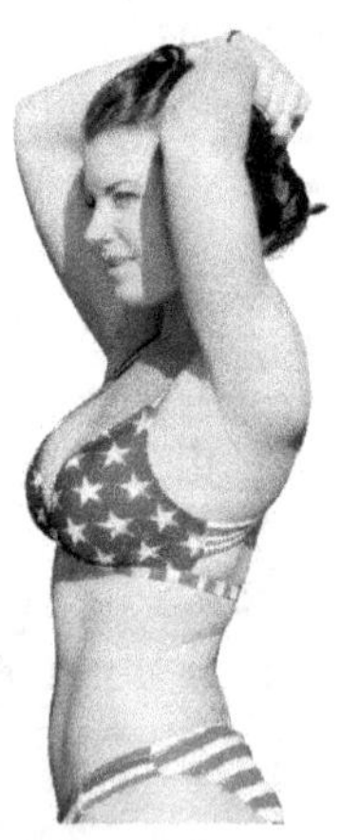

Benefits of waxing for summer

The following are some advantages of waxing that make it a great summertime hair removal option:

1. Long-Lasting Effects: Hair is removed from the root during waxing, producing effects that may endure for several weeks. This means you won't need to do touch-ups frequently to maintain your smooth, hair-free skin throughout the summer.

2. Regrowth that is scarce: After waxing, hair frequently grows back softer and finer, which makes it less obvious and more comfortable in between waxing treatments.

3. Skin that is even and smooth: In addition to removing hair, waxing also exfoliates the skin, giving it a smoother, more uniform texture. This is very useful for getting a faultless appearance in swimwear and other summer clothing.

4. Lessening of ingrown hairs: Waxing pulls hair from the root, preventing ingrown hairs, unlike shaving, which can cause them. As a result, fewer pimples and irritation are produced, improving the appearance.

5. Efficiency: Waxing can cover larger regions in a single session and can be completed rather quickly. It is therefore a quick choice, ideal for those hectic summer days.

6. Positivity for Beach and Pool Activities: You can comfortably partake in water sports, sunbathing, and beach vacations with waxed skin without worrying about noticeable stubble or razor burns.

7. Less Maintenance: Waxing requires fewer maintenance sessions than regular shaving. This gives you more time to take advantage of your summertime experiences.

8. Preventive Measures: Waxing helps you keep healthy, comfortable skin throughout the summer by lowering the chance of skin irritation and razor burn that can come from routine shaving.

9. Enhanced Tan: Smooth, exfoliated skin as a result of waxing can make your tan more even and attractive, boosting your summer glow.

10. Various Applications: The bikini line, legs, arms, and underarms are just a few locations that can be waxed to get a smooth appearance that matches your summer fashion.

Waxing can improve your overall experience by giving you a carefree and confident way to take full advantage of the activities that the season has to offer. Include waxing in your summer grooming routine.

Safety precautions

To ensure a pleasant and secure experience when waxing your bikini line at home, it's important to follow a few safety precautions:

1. A patch test: To check for any allergic responses to the waxing product or unpleasant effects, perform a patch test on a tiny patch of skin. In order to ensure there is no irritation, wait 24 hours.

2. Dry and clean skin: To avoid infections, start with clean, dry skin. Before waxing, wash the area with mild soap and water.

3. Hygiene: To reduce the possibility of introducing bacteria, make sure your hands, the waxing instruments, and the work space are clean.

4. Temperature Check: Before using the wax on your skin, check the wax's temperature. It should be comfortable—warm but not sweltering. Always adhere to the manufacturer's heating instructions.

5. Stay away from sunburned skin: Sunburned or newly tanned skin should not be waxed since it may be more sensitive and vulnerable to harm.

6. Drugs and disorders: Consult a healthcare provider before waxing if you are taking any drugs or have skin disorders like eczema or psoriasis.

7. Hair Length: Make sure your hair is long enough to be waxed effectively, which is usually between 1/4 and 1/2 inch (6 and 12 millimeters).

8. Exfoliation: Exfoliation should be avoided before waxing because it can make your skin more sensitive and prone to irritation.

9. Prevention of Irritation: To prevent irritation, wait at least 24 hours after waxing to use perfumes, lotions, or other fragranced products on the area that has been waxed.

10. Apply Light Pressure: After waxing, apply light pressure to the area to soothe it. For the first 24 hours, stay away from activities that could create friction or tight clothes.

11. No Double Dipping: To prevent contaminating the wax with bacteria, never use the same waxing applicator for more than one application.

12. Sun Protection: If you intend to spend time in the sun, apply sunscreen to the waxed area. Skin that has just been waxed may be more vulnerable to UV radiation.

13. Avoid hot tubs or swimming pools: For at least 24 hours after waxing, avoid swimming in chlorinated pools or hot tubs to avoid irritation.

14. Consult a specialist: Consider seeking advice from a licenced esthetician or choosing to have a professional waxing session if you have sensitive skin or are unsure about the procedure.

Prioritizing these safety measures will help you to establish a relaxing and risk-free environment for your at-home bikini line waxing procedure, giving you the assurance you need to attain smooth, summer-ready skin.

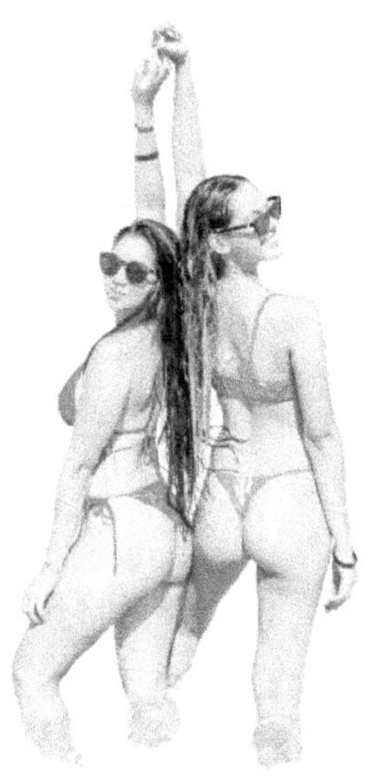

Chapter 2

Gathering Supplies

List of required waxing supplies

The following tools and supplies are required for a successful and comfortable bikini line waxing experience at home:

1. Waxing Kit: Invest in a good waxing set that comes with strips, tools, and wax. Both soft wax and hard wax kits are offered.

2. Wax: Depending on your preferences and skin type, select either hard wax or soft wax. While soft wax is adaptable for broader areas, hard wax is suited for delicate areas like the bikini line.

3. Wax Warmer: If you're using hard wax, a wax warmer is necessary to melt the wax to the right temperature. Make sure the temperature can be adjusted.

4. The applicants: For applying the wax, get wooden or disposable applicators. They come in different sizes and shapes to fit different spaces.

5. Waxing Strips: You will need cloth or paper waxing strips for removal if you're using soft wax. These are frequently present in waxing kits.

6. Use a pre-wax cleaner: To make sure the area is clean and free of sweat, oils, and lotions before waxing.

7. Talcum Oil or Powder: Talcum powder or oil can be used to protect the skin and improve the adhesion of the wax.

8. Post-Waxing Lotion or Oil: After waxing, a calming oil or lotion helps to soothe the skin and remove any leftover wax. Seek out products made especially for aftercare.

9. Antiseptic Wipes: To lower the risk of infection, clean the region with antiseptic wipes before waxing.

10. Tweezers: Have tweezers on standby in case you need to make precise touch-ups.

11. Mirror: Using a wall-mounted or handheld mirror will help you apply makeup correctly by allowing you to see the area properly.

12. Cotton Pads or Cloth: To remove extra oil, wax, or residue, keep cotton pads or a clean cloth handy.

13. Aloe gel or an ice pack: After waxing, an ice pack or aloe vera gel can help ease any skin redness or soreness.

14. Gloves: To maintain cleanliness and stop the spread of bacteria, use disposable gloves.

15. Keep a trash bag: Trash bags should be kept close, so that you can easily throw away used waxing strips and applicators.

16. Scissors or a Hair Trimmer: Before waxing, if required, reduce hair to the proper length using a trimmer or scissors.

Read the directions that come with your selected waxing kit and tools before you start. A successful, efficient, and comfortable bikini line waxing session at home will be made possible by having all the required supplies on hand.

Recommended types of wax

The appropriate kind of wax must be used while waxing the bikini line in order to provide results that are both efficient and comfortable. Hard wax and soft wax are the two major types of wax frequently used for at-home waxing. Each style has particular advantages and things to think about:

1. Hard Wax: Appropriate for Sensitive Areas Because it sticks to the hair rather than the skin, hard wax is frequently advised for delicate areas like the bikini line. This lessens the possibility of pulling on sensitive skin.

Less Hurting: Hard wax is typically easier to remove than soft wax because it hardens as it cools and can be scraped off without using strips.

Hair that is shorter: Hard wax is great for touch-ups in between sessions since it can remove shorter hair lengths effectively.

Reduced Irritation Risk: Hard wax has the potential to be kinder and less abrasive because it doesn't adhere to the skin as much.

2. Soft Wax : "Variable for Larger Areas" For larger areas like the arms, chest, and legs, soft wax is more adaptable. It may cover a larger area quickly

Works Best on Coarse Hair Soft wax may be able to grab and remove your hair more effectively if it is coarser.

Waxing Strips Required: Waxing strips are used to remove a small coating of soft wax after application. For larger areas, this approach might be faster.

Bonus for exfoliation Additionally, when the skin is removed by a soft wax, it exfoliates, making the skin smoother.

The decision between hard wax and soft wax ultimately comes down to your level of comfort, hair type, and preferences. Due to its gentleness on sensitive skin, many people favor using hard wax for the bikini line. Always adhere to the waxing kit's instructions and carry out a patch test to make sure the wax is compatible with your skin type.

Preparing your workspace

For a good and relaxing bikini line waxing session, setting up a clean and organized workspace is crucial. How to set up your workplace is as follows:

1. Select an Appropriate Location: Choose a spot that is tidy and well-lit so you can comfortably wax yourself. For greater vision, a bathroom with a mirror is preferable.

2. Cover the area: To Prevent wax drips and spills by laying down washable or disposable towels or sheets. This facilitates cleanup.

3. Set up your waxing kit: Setting up a waxing kit should include the wax warmer (if using hard wax), wax, applicators, and waxing strips. Make sure everything is accessible.

4. Collect Supplies: A pre-wax cleaner, talcum powder or oil, post-waxing oil or lotion, antiseptic wipes, a pair of tweezers, and calming goods for after waxing should all be placed close by.

5. Clean the region: Use a mild pre-wax cleaner to remove any oils, lotions, or sweat from the area you intend to wax. To dry the area, use a clean towel.

6. Heat the wax: If you're using hard wax, switch on the wax warmer and warm the wax as directed by the maker. Before applying the temperature to your skin, always test it first.

7. Check the consistency and temperature: Make sure the wax has reached the proper consistency and is at a comfortable temperature. Spreadability is ideal, but not too much runniness.

8. Wash your hands: Wear disposable gloves and wash your hands properly as a matter of hygiene.

9. Prepare the Skin: If desired, lightly dust the skin with talcum powder or oil to protect it and help the wax cling.

10. Have A Mirror: Position the mirror so that you can easily view the area you are waxing. As a result, the application and removal are precise.

11. Garbage Bag: For simple disposal of old waxing strips and applicators, have a small trash bag close by.

12. Play Calming Music or Create a Relaxing atmosphere. This will help you remain relaxed and at ease throughout the procedure.

12. Ventilation: Make sure the room has enough ventilation if you're using any products with intense scents.

14. Test Your Technique: Before beginning the entire procedure, practice putting wax on and taking it off from a tiny area to become accustomed to the technique.

You'll be able to concentrate on the waxing procedure and get better results by creating a tidy and organized workspace. Remain serene and tranquil at all times because a laid-back attitude can help make your bikini line waxing experience more successful.

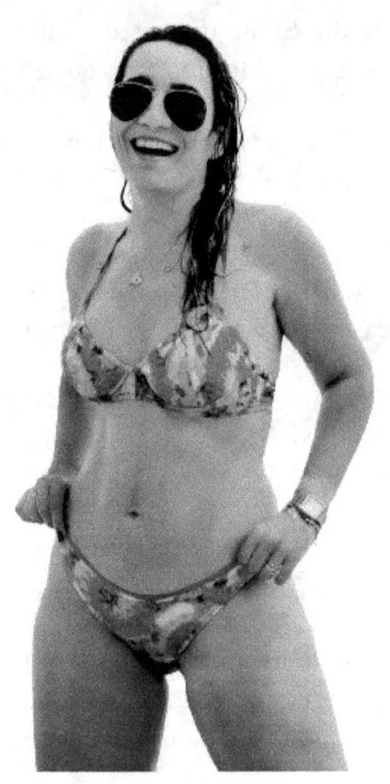

Chapter 3

Preparing Your Skin

Exfoliating and cleansing

Before waxing, the bikini area must be properly exfoliated and cleansed to ensure efficient hair removal and reduce the risk of irritation. For the best exfoliation and cleanliness, adhere to these steps:

1. **Time:** 24 to 48 hours before your scheduled waxing appointment, exfoliate the region. This provides time for your skin to heal from any potential discomfort caused by exfoliation.

2. **Gentle Exfoliation:** To remove dead skin cells from the surface, use a body brush or a mild exfoliating scrub. Exfoliation makes the wax more adherent and helps prevent ingrown hairs.

3. **Warm Water:** Use warm water to open up your pores prior to exfoliation. This softens the hair follicles and increases the efficiency of exfoliation.

4. **Be gentle :** Use gentle circular motions to gently massage the exfoliant into the skin. The bikini area is sensitive, so don't scrub too hard.

5. Rinse Completely: After exfoliating, thoroughly rinse the area with warm water to get rid of any exfoliant residue.

6. Cleaning : Use a moderate, fragrance-free soap or cleanser to clean the bikini area. Use mild chemicals or perfumes; harsh chemicals and strong fragrances might irritate the skin.

7. Pat Dry: Apply a clean, soft towel to the area and gently pat it dry. Avoid rubbing because doing so can aggravate the skin even more.

8. No lotions or oils: Before waxing, avoid using any creams, lotions, or oils on the region. These may act as a barrier, preventing the wax from effectively sticking.

9. Look for irritation: After exfoliation and washing, it is preferable to wait until your skin has fully healed before scheduling a waxing appointment if you experience any redness, inflammation, or irritation.

Cleansing and exfoliating properly prepare the skin for waxing by ensuring that the wax adheres effectively to the hair and lowering the risk of ingrown hairs or discomfort. Everybody has varied skin, so if you have sensitive skin, be extra gentle when exfoliating to prevent needless irritability.

Trimming hair to the appropriate length

Before waxing, hair should be properly trimmed to the desired length for a smoother, more efficient waxing procedure. To prepare for waxing the bikini line, trim the hair as follows:

1. Consider Hair Length: Your hair's length should be checked. The ideal hair length for waxing is between 6 and 12 mm, or around 1/4 to 1/2 inch. Trimming it is a good idea if it is longer than this.

2. Trimming Equipment: Use tiny, razor-sharp scissors or a hair trimmer made especially for delicate areas. Make sure the tools are sanitized and clean.

3. Brush or comb the hair: Brush or comb the hair in the bikini area to make sure it is straight and flat against the skin. This facilitates a cleaner trim.

4. Start Gently: Start trimming by taking off a little bit of hair at a time. Trimming too much by accident is preferable to trimming too little at first.

5. Evenly Trim: Trim the hair uniformly while maintaining a parallel grip on the scissors or trimmer. To prevent nicks, be cautious while cutting too close to the skin.

6. Keep the Shape: If you have a particular shape or style in mind (for example, a particular bikini line style), stick to that shape when trimming.

7. Check the hair always: Remember that you can always cut more hair if necessary, but once it has been chopped, it cannot be grown back.

8. Avoid trimming too much: To avoid making waxing more difficult and maybe painful, don't trim your hair too short.

9. Gently Brush Again: After trimming, gently brush or comb the hair one more time to make sure it is straight and evenly distributed.

10. Clean Up: Properly dispose of the hair that has been cut and clean the trimming equipment.

Trimming the hair to the proper length before waxing can help ensure that the wax adheres to the hair efficiently. If you're not sure how much to cut, you can let it sit a little longer because the wax will still hold the hair and work well.

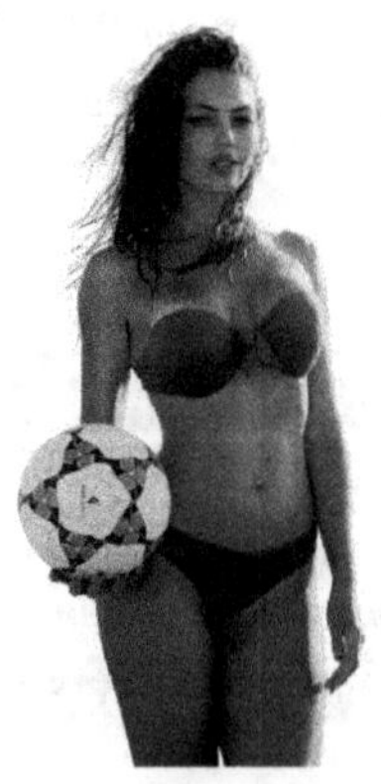

Skin sensitivity consideration

It's important to consider how sensitive your skin is before bikini line waxing. Here are some things to keep in mind to make waxing safe and comfortable:

1. A patch test: Apply a tiny bit of wax to a small section of your bikini line to conduct a patch test before waxing. Check for any unfavorable reactions, such as redness, irritability, or itching, after 24 hours.

2. Choose the Right Wax: If you are aware that your skin is prone to irritation or redness, choose a wax that is designed for sensitive skin.

3. Allergies to skin: It is advisable to speak with a dermatologist before waxing if you have a history of skin allergies or sensitivities. They can give advice on probable allergens and suggest suitable goods.

4. Prevent Sunburn: Sunburned or recently tanned skin should not be waxed as it may be more sensitive and vulnerable to harm.

5. Medications: Some drugs, like blood thinners or retinoids, can make your skin more sensitive. If you use such medications, talk to a healthcare provider before waxing.

6. The menstrual cycle : For some people, the menstrual cycle makes their skin more sensitive. If this is the case for you, think about changing the time of your waxing appointment.

7. Avoid using harsh chemicals: Applying chemicals like exfoliants, retinoids, or chemical peels on the bikini area a few days before waxing should be avoided because they may make the skin more sensitive.

8. Cooling Preparations: A day or two before waxing, some people find that applying a relaxing aloe vera gel or calming lotion will help the skin become ready.

9. Seek Professional Advice: Consider getting your waxing done by a licensed esthetician if you have very sensitive skin or have previously experienced negative reactions to waxing.

10. Pay Attention to Your Skin: Discuss your discomfort and consider interrupting the waxing operation if you feel any stinging, pain, or discomfort. Your happiness and comfort come first.

Keep in mind that each person's skin is unique. A smoother and more comfortable bikini line waxing procedure can be achieved by being aware of your skin's sensitivity and making the necessary preparations. It's always a good idea to begin with a patch test if you're unsure and build up to a complete waxing session gradually.

Chapter 4

Steps for Bikini Line Waxing

Applying Talcum powder or oil for the protection

Before waxing, talcum powder or oil can be applied as a preventative precaution to make the process smoother and more comfortable. Here is how to employ each choice:

1. Talcum Powder: Use baby powder or talcum powder designed especially for delicate skin, as these are less likely to irritate skin.

Apply a little layer of talcum powder to the bikini area. This makes it easier for the wax to stick to the hair by absorbing extra moisture, oils, and sweat.

Before putting on the wax, gently pat the area to get rid of any extra powder.

2. Oil: Choose a mild, non-comedogenic oil like jojoba oil, coconut oil, or olive oil if you're using oil as a moisturizer. Avoid oils with strong scents or textures that could irritate or clog pores.

Massage a small amount of oil into the bikini region. By creating a barrier between the wax and your skin, this can lessen pain.

Avoid using too much oil because it can make it difficult for the wax to adhere to the hair properly.

To prevent the wax from clinging to your skin and creating unnecessary agony, use talcum powder or oil as a barrier between the wax and your skin. Feel free to experiment with both approaches to determine which one suits your skin type and preferences the best. Just a small layer of powder or oil should be applied to avoid interfering with the waxing procedure.

Heating and testing the wax temperature

To achieve a secure and comfortable bikini line waxing procedure, the wax must be heated to the proper temperature and tested before being applied to your skin. To heat the wax and gauge its temperature, follow these steps:

1. **Read Instructions:** To correctly heat the wax, first read the manufacturer's instructions. It's possible that different varieties of wax have different temperature requirements.

2. **Wax Warmer:** Use a wax warmer made specifically for hard wax if you're using one. Soft wax is frequently sold in packages that can be heated directly in the microwave.

3. **Low to Medium Setting:** Lower or raise the wax warmer temperature. Avoid using excessive heat because it might cause overheating and skin burns.

4. Check consistency: The wax should melt into a creamy, smooth consistency as it warms up. To achieve equal heating, occasionally stir the wax.

5. Safety Precautions: Be careful when handling hot wax or waxing equipment, and never leave the wax heating alone.

6. Testing Temperature: To check the temperature, place a tiny drop of wax on the inside of your wrist. Similar to the bikini line, this area of your skin is delicate. The wax shouldn't be uncomfortably hot, just warm. Wait for it to get a little bit cooler if it's too hot before continuing.

7 Wait for the ideal temperature: Allow the wax to cool for a few minutes if it is too hot. Working with slightly cooler wax is preferable to running the risk of skin burning.

8. Changing the Temperature: You might need to gently reheat the wax if it becomes very thick from cooling down too much. Avoid overheating because it might cause burns on the skin.

9. Stirring: Before putting the wax on, give it one last stir to make sure it is uniformly warm and thick.

You should always test the wax's temperature on a small patch of delicate skin before using it on your bikini line to prevent pain or burns. Wax that has been heated properly should spread evenly, stick to the hair, and be comfortable against your skin.

Applying wax in small sections

When waxing your bikini line, the key to precise and effective hair removal is to apply the wax in small parts. This is how you do it:

1. Divide the Area: "Divide the Area" means to divide the bikini area into more manageable chunks. This enables you to work methodically and guarantees that each region gets the attention it needs.

2. Applicator: Dip the wooden stick-shaped wax applicator into the hot wax. To ensure that the wax covers one side of the stick equally, hold the applicator at an angle.

3. Apply the wax: In one area of the bikini area, apply a thin coating of wax in the direction of hair growth. Just 2 to 3 inches broad should be your starting point.

4. Avoid Overlapping: Take care not to apply wax to regions that have already had waxing, as this can irritate the skin and result in unneeded pain.

5. Smooth Application: Use a smooth, even application of the wax to ensure that it sticks to the hairs. For simple removal, the wax should be thicker in the middle and thinner on the borders.

6. Press Waxing Strip: If using soft wax, cover the applied wax right away with a waxing strip. To make sure the strip adheres to the wax, press down hard.

7. Rub the strip: To help the waxing strip stick to the wax and hair, gently rub it a few times. This guarantees a secure hold for efficient hair removal.

8. Hold the Skin Tight: Using your free hand, tighten the skin around the waxed area. This lessens the pain experienced during the wax removal procedure.

9. Quick Pull: For best results, quickly pull the waxing strip off in the direction that the hair grows, keeping the strip close to the skin.

10. Repeat the procedure: Continue to apply wax in little pieces as you work your way across the bikini area. Always remember to apply wax in the direction that the hair grows.

11. Verify Accuracy: After waxing each part, look for any hairs that may have remained. Reapply wax as necessary, then shave off any residual hair.

You can better manage the process and make sure that each region is fully treated by applying wax in small chunks. By concentrating on smaller locations at a time, this approach also reduces discomfort. Keep in mind that for results that are smooth and hair-free, patience and accuracy are essential.

Placing wax strips and removal techniques

For effective and comfortable hair removal along the bikini line, use the right removal methods and wax strip placement. This is how you do it:

1. Placing the Wax Strips:

1. Place a waxing strip over the targeted area as soon as a thin coating of wax has been applied. To make sure the strip sticks to the wax, press down hard.

2. Ensure that the strip provides a hold for simple removal by sticking out just a little bit beyond the waxed region.

3. Rub the strip a few times if you're using soft wax to help it stick to the wax and hair.

2. Wax Removal Methods:

1. With one hand, keep the skin taut around the area where the waxing strip will be applied. This eases irritation and facilitates the wax removal procedure.

2. Quick Pull: Grab the end of the waxed strip that is not attached to the skin with your other hand. Pull the strip off in the opposite direction of hair growth in a single fast stroke, keeping the strip parallel to the skin.

3. Pulling Direction: Pull the strip back parallel to the skin and just below the skin's surface when removing it. This lessens discomfort and makes hair removal more efficient.

4. Hold Your Breath: Inhale deeply before removing the strip, then quickly exhale as you do so. This can lessen some of the discomfort experienced during the procedure.

5. Repeat the Procedure: Use the removal method, strips, and wax on each portion of the bikini area as necessary.

6. Handling Residue: You can use a post-waxing oil or the edge of a fresh waxing strip to carefully remove any leftover wax from the skin after removing the waxing strip.

7. Prevent double-dipping by not recycling wax strips. To ensure the best grip and prevent transferring wax to areas that have already been waxed, use a fresh strip for each removal.

Keep in mind that using the right removal methods is essential to minimizing pain and removing hair effectively. Start with smaller regions and progress to larger ones if you're new to waxing or find it uncomfortable. The process will get easier and more effective as you become acclimated to the feel and technique.

Chapter 5

After Care

Removing residual wax and soothing the skin

It's crucial to take action to remove any remaining wax and calm the skin around the bikini area after removing the waxing strips. This is how you do it:

1. Eliminating Remaining Wax:

1. Post-Waxing: Oil Using a cotton pad or cloth, apply a post-waxing oil. Any spots with leftover wax should be gently rubbed with the oil. The oil aids in the wax's disintegration and facilitates its removal.

2. Gentle Scratching: Apply the oil to the skin by rubbing it in moderate circular motions. Because the skin around the bikini area might be sensitive, avoid applying undue pressure.

3. Repeat as necessary: If there is still wax left behind, use more oil and rub gently until all traces of the wax are gone.

2. Calming the Skin

1. Cool Compress: For a few minutes, apply a cold compress or a cool, moist towel to the waxed area. This can help calm any irritation and lessen redness.

2. Post-Waxing Cream: Utilize a post-waxing lotion created especially to calm and soothe the skin after hair removal. Look for products that have chamomile or aloe vera as an ingredient.

3. Aloe Vera Gel: Pure aloe vera gel can be applied to the skin to soothe it and lessen redness. Use aloe vera without alcohol or added scents.

4. Wear breathable clothing: Loose-fitting clothing after waxing to prevent rubbing and irritation on the newly waxed skin.

5. Avoid Heat and Irritants: For the following 24-48 hours after waxing, stay away from hot baths, saunas, sunbathing, and activities that could create friction or excessive perspiration.

6. No Sun Exposure: Apply sunscreen to any waxed areas of your body that will be exposed to the sun to shield the delicate skin from UV rays.

7. Hydrate: Drink lots of water to keep your skin moisturized from the inside out and hasten healing.

These techniques will help you remove any remaining wax and effectively soothe your skin after waxing. You can enjoy the effects of your waxing session and a comfortable recovery by treating your skin delicately and with care in the post-waxing phase.

Applying post waxing products

To relax and care for your skin after a bikini line waxing treatment, post-waxing creams must be applied. The best way to apply post-waxing products is as follows:

1. Cleanse the Area: After removing any remaining wax, gently scrub the waxed area with a mild, fragrance-free cleanser to get rid of any oil or debris that may have remained.

2. Pat Dry: Apply a clean, soft towel to the area and gently pat it dry. As the skin may be sensitive after waxing, refrain from rubbing.

3. Post-Waxing Oil or Lotion: Pick a post-waxing oil or lotion that is designed specifically to calm and soothe the skin after hair removal.
Use your fingertips to apply a tiny amount of the product to the waxed region and gently rub it in a circular motion.
Pay close attention as you massage the substance into your skin until it is completely absorbed.

4. Aloe Vera Gel: Aloe vera gel in its purest form can be applied to the skin to calm it if you choose a natural remedy. Make sure there are no additional scents or alcohols in it.
To remove wax, use a small coating of aloe vera gel and gently rub it in until it disappears.

5. Steer clear of fragrances: For at least 24 hours after waxing, it is advised to avoid using perfumes, scented lotions, or other items with strong odors on the waxed area because they may irritate the skin.

6. Repeat as necessary: If you suffer any discomfort, redness, or irritation throughout the day, you can reapply post-waxing treatments.

7. Avoid Touching the region: After using the post-waxing product, keep your hands off the waxed region unless absolutely necessary to avoid spreading bacteria and irritating the skin.

8. Wear Loose Clothing: To reduce friction and promote proper airflow for the skin, dress in loose-fitting, breathable clothing.

9. Maintaining hydration: This will help your skin heal more quickly. Drink plenty of water.

Products for use after waxing help calm the skin, lessen redness, and lessen any potential discomfort or irritability. Select items that are soft, hypoallergenic, and appropriate for skin that is sensitive. To ensure a comfortable recovery, pay attention to your skin's response and modify your post-waxing routine as necessary.

Applying certain activities and products

To guarantee the comfort of your skin and avoid potential irritation or issues, there are some activities and items you should avoid for a while after a bikini line waxing treatment. Here is a list of things to avoid:

Activities to Avoid Include:

1. Saunas and hot baths For at least 24 to 48 hours after waxing, stay away from hot baths, saunas, steam rooms, and hot tubs. Heat can aggravate newly waxed skin and raise the possibility of infection.

2. Excessive Sweating: Excessive sweating can irritate the skin and produce discomfort while engaged in vigorous exercises or other activities. For the first day or two, choose easy activities.

3. Avoid prolonged sun exposure to the area that has been waxed for at least 24 hours. Freshly waxed skin is more susceptible to sunburn since it is more UV-sensitive.

4. Swimming: For at least 24 hours after waxing, avoid swimming in chlorinated pools, seas, or hot tubs. Both saltwater and chlorine can irritate the skin.

5. Tannining: After waxing, wait at least 24 hours before using self-tanning creams or tanning beds. The skin may become irritated and discolored after tanning.

6. Avoid harsh exfoliants or exfoliating scrubs on the waxed region for at least 48 hours after waxing. Exfoliation may make the skin even more sensitive.

Products to evade:

1. Fragrances and Fragrant Products For at least 24 hours, refrain from using perfumes, scented lotions, and other products with potent scents on the waxed region. Freshly waxed skin can become inflamed by fragrances.

2. Retinoids and chemical peels: For a few days after waxing, refrain from using products that contain chemical exfoliants like AHAs, BHAs, and retinoids. These might irritate others.

3. Medications for topical acne Avoid using any acne treatments with benzoyl peroxide, salicylic acid, or other active chemicals on the waxed region.

4. Deodorants containing aluminium Deodorants containing aluminium should be avoided for at least 24 hours after waxing your underarms since they may irritate the area.

It's important to keep in mind that every person's skin reacts differently, so it's wise to exercise caution and pay attention to your skin's needs. Give your skin some time to heal if you notice any redness, irritation, or discomfort before returning to your regular routine or using certain products.

Tips for preventing ingrown hair

After bikini line waxing, maintaining smooth, healthy skin requires taking steps to prevent ingrown hairs. Here are some suggestions to reduce the likelihood of ingrown hairs:

1. Exfoliate regularly: To eliminate dead skin cells and prevent hair from getting tangled under the skin, gently exfoliate the bikini area using a moderate exfoliating scrub or a soft brush.

2. Exfoliate the region before waxing: Do this a day or two beforehand. With any ingrown hairs lifted closer to the surface, waxing can more easily remove them.

3. Employ the appropriate exfoliation method: Exfoliating should be done gently. Avoid using aggressive scrubbers because they might aggravate ingrown hairs and irritate the skin.

4. Avoid Wearing Tight Clothes: After waxing, put on loose-fitting clothing to reduce friction and let the skin breathe. Hair could curl back into the skin when wearing restrictive garments.

5. Moisturize Regularly: Use a mild, non-comedogenic lotion to keep the skin hydrated. Ingrown hairs are less likely to appear on moisturized skin.

6. Refrain from touching or picking at the waxed region because doing so might spread bacteria and cause ingrown hairs.

7. Use a Soft Brush: After the initial period of healing, you can gently exfoliate the region during your routine showers using a soft brush or exfoliating gloves.

8. Do not shave in between appointments: Shaving can make ingrown hairs more likely since shaving makes hair tips sharper and more easily penetrate the skin.

9. Routine Waxing: By weakening the hair follicles and decreasing their capacity to curl back into the skin, regular waxing treatments can aid in the prevention of ingrown hairs.

10. Address Early Warning Signs: Avoid picking at any red pimples or indications of ingrown hairs. Instead, use a warm compress or a light exfoliating product to aid in releasing the hair.

11. Choose the Right Wax: Choose waxing services provided by skilled estheticians or professionals since they have the knowledge to reduce the risk of ingrown hairs.

12. Seek advice from a dermatologist: Consider seeing a dermatologist for individualized advice and treatment options if you frequently experience painful ingrown hairs or have a history of skin problems.

You may lessen the possibility of ingrown hairs and benefit from smooth, hair-free skin after bikini line waxing by adhering to these suggestions and maintaining a regular skincare routine.

Chapter 6

Troubleshooting

Dealing with pain and discomfort

It's typical to feel uncomfortable and in pain after getting your bikini line waxed, especially if it's your first time or if you have sensitive skin. Here are some methods to efficiently manage your pain and discomfort:

1. Painkillers available over-the-counter: In order to lessen pain and discomfort, you can take an over-the-counter painkiller like ibuprofen or acetaminophen before waxing. Observe the dose recommendations.

2. Cool Compress: For a few minutes, apply a cool compress or a damp, cool cloth to the waxed region. This can ease irritation and soothe the skin, as well as lessen redness.

3. Pure aloe vera gel: Pure aloe vera gel should be applied to the area that has been waxed. Aloe vera contains calming qualities that might lessen discomfort and irritability.

4. Apply post-waxing products: Apply products that are made specifically to relax and calm the skin. These products can aid in reducing discomfort and accelerating healing.

5. Loose Clothes: To reduce friction and allow the skin to breathe, dress comfortably in loose-fitting clothing made of breathable materials. Wearing uncomfortable clothing can make it worse.

6. Avoid Hot Water: For the first 24 hours after waxing, stay away from hot showers, baths, or steam rooms because the heat can make you feel more uncomfortable and irritated.

7. Hydrolysis: To stay hydrated, sip lots of water. Skin that is properly hydrated is more robust and recovers more rapidly.

8. Distraction: Take part in activities that take your mind off your discomfort, like reading a book, watching a movie, or listening to music.

9. Use relaxation strategies: Strategies such as deep breathing, meditation, or other methods should be used to manage discomfort and reduce stress.

10. Avoid touching: Keep your hands off the waxed area to prevent irritation and discomfort from escalating.

11. Time: After waxing, discomfort usually goes away within a day or two as your skin adjusts and heals.

12. Seek Professional Advice: Ask a dermatologist or esthetician for help if you have chronic pain, severe redness, or symptoms of an allergic reaction.

In particular, if it's your first time, keep in mind that any soreness you experience after waxing is typically temporary and normal. With each subsequent appointment, you might notice that the discomfort decreases as you get used to waxing.

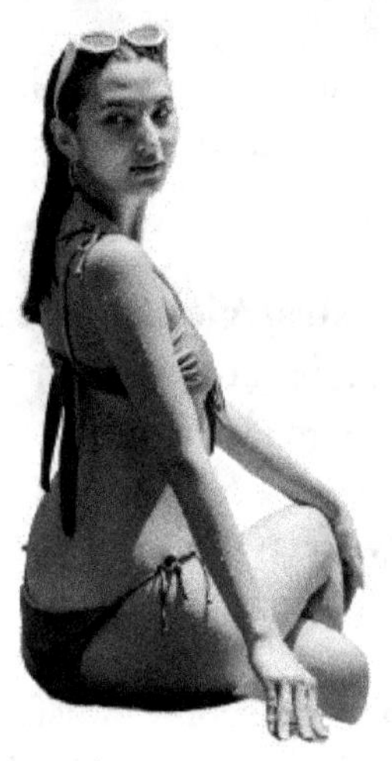

Chapter 7

Maintenance and Upkeep

Frequency of Bikini waxing

Based on individual characteristics such as hair growth rate, hair texture, and personal preferences, the frequency of bikini waxing can change. However, there are a few general recommendations to take into account when deciding how frequently to get a bikini wax:

1. The Hair Growth Cycle: The usual length of a hair growth cycle is 3 to 6 weeks. Therefore, a few weeks after waxing, you might start to see regrowth in the bikini area.

2. Individual Hair Growth Rate: Take note of how soon your hair regrows. Perhaps some people heal more fast than others

3. Maintenance Waxing: Many women want to get a bikini wax every 4 to 6 weeks for consistent smoothness. This timeline fits with the typical cycle of hair growth.

4. Regular Upkeep: Over time, frequent waxing may cause the hair to thin and become sparser. You might discover that, as a result, you require fewer waxing sessions.

5. Special times: Some people decide to get a wax before important events, vacations, or other times where they want to look good and be hair-free.

6. Skin Sensitivity: Waiting a little bit longer between waxing appointments if you have sensitive skin may help prevent rashes.

7. Hair Length: Before your next waxing treatment, make sure your hair is the appropriate length (usually 1/4 to 1/2 inch). This enables the wax to effectively grasp the hair.

8. Prevent Over-Waxing: Waxing should not be done too frequently since this might result in increased skin sensitivity, discomfort, or ingrown hairs.

9 Skin sensitivity: Depending on your hair type, skin sensitivity, and personal preferences, see a professional esthetician to determine the optimal waxing regimen.

You must keep in mind that the best waxing frequency is specific to you. Observe how your skin responds after each session, then alter the timing as necessary. Regular waxing can assist in preserving smoother skin over time, but make sure to give your skin time to heal between treatments.

Alternatives hair removal methods

Bikini line waxing is not the only hair removal option to take into account. Every technique has pros and cons of its own. Here are a few well-liked substitutes:

1. Shaving: Shaving is a simple and quick technique. But because hair regrows so quickly, stubble may develop. Additionally, it's critical to use caution to prevent nicks and discomfort.

2. Depilatory Creams: These lotions remove hair from the skin's surface. They are simple to use, but they smell strongly, and they might not be good for skin that is sensitive.

3. Epilation: Epilators are machines that pull hair out from the root mechanically to remove it. Shaving might produce results that last longer, but it can also be painful and result in short-term redness.

4. Laser Hair Removal: To stop hair growth, laser treatments target hair follicles. Although it frequently requires numerous sessions, it is more long-term. It is advised to seek professional treatment for the best outcomes.

5. Electrolysis: Electrical currents are used in electrolysis to kill hair follicles. Permanent hair removal can be accomplished with it, although it can take a while and be uncomfortable.

6. Threading: To remove hair, threading requires twisting a thread. Although it can be more uncomfortable, it is precise and suited for small areas like the brows.

7. Sugaring: Similar to waxing, sugaring removes hair by applying a paste made of sugar. It is thought to be kinder to the skin and may cause less discomfort.

8. Cream depilation: Applying a cream that dissolves hair at the skin's surface is known as cream depilation. Although it is simple to apply, it can have a strong odour, and some people may find it irritating.

9. Home Laser Hair Removal: IPL (intense pulsed light) technology is used in some at-home hair removal equipment. Because results can differ, it's critical to carefully follow directions.

Consider aspects including your tolerance for pain, skin sensitivity, hair texture, and desired duration of results when selecting an alternate hair removal treatment. Before attempting a new technique, it's a good idea to do some research and even speak with an expert to see which will be most effective for you.

Tips for smoother results over time

Regardless of the method you select, follow these suggestions to gradually get smoother and more effective hair removal results:

1. Consistency: Adhere to a consistent hair removal regimen. Regular care, whether you wax, shave, or use another technique, keeps your skin smoother.

2. Exfoliation: Performing regular exfoliation keeps your skin smooth and prevents ingrown hairs. A few times per week, gently exfoliate; however, avoid over-exfoliating since this might irritate the skin.

3. Hydrolysis: Utilize moisturizers and drink lots of water to keep your skin moisturized. Skin that has been properly hydrated is less irritable and more supple.

4. Use proper instrument : Use the proper instruments for the hair removal approach you've chosen. This covers high-quality epilators, waxing kits, and razors.

5. Hair Growth Length: Check that the length of your hair is adequate for the technique you're applying. For optimal results, hair should be between 1/4 and 1/2 inch long before waxing.

6. Professional Assistance: For the greatest results, seek expert guidance and treatment if you're thinking about more permanent hair removal techniques like laser hair removal or electrolysis.

7. Avoid Irritants: Prevent irritation by avoiding strong soaps, perfumed products, and tight garments right after shaving.

8. Products for Post-Hair Removal: Use post-hair removal solutions to soothe the skin and lessen irritability, such as calming lotions or aloe vera gel.

9. Sun Protection: Avoid exposing your skin to the sun, especially right after shaving. To avoid sunburn and hyperpigmentation, wear sunscreen.

10. Patience: It could take some time to get results that are consistently smooth, especially when switching between methods. Let your skin acclimatize before touching it.

11. Prevent Over-Treating: Over-treating your skin can irritate it and cause harm. Observe the instructions provided for each hair removal technique.

12. Consult with experts: Consult a dermatologist or esthetician for advice if you're unclear about the best course of action for your skin or are having ongoing problems.

Keep in mind that each person's skin is unique. To find the regimen and products that work best for you, some trial and error may be necessary. You'll eventually be able to get smoother and more satisfying hair removal outcomes if you're patient and mindful of your skin's requirements.

Conclusion

This book has given you a thorough understanding on perfecting the art of at-home waxing for the summer, which will help you attain delightfully smooth skin and confidently flaunt your bikini line. You've gathered a lot of knowledge to design a customized hair removal programme that meets your tastes and skin type, from the significance of grooming to the painstaking procedures of preparation, application, and aftercare.

Consider the adage "practice makes perfect" as you embark on your hair removal adventure. Accept the craft of waxing with patience and accuracy, making each session a step towards having hair-free skin as well as an increase in your self-confidence. You are prepared to face bikini season head-on with the advice, strategies, and insights provided in these pages, feeling confident and prepared to take on the world.

May your trip be one of easy outcomes, little discomfort, and a fresh appreciation for the beauty that comes with well-kept bikini lines. As you start down this path of self-care and confidence, keep in mind that the secret to success isn't just in the method but also in the inner-radiating self-assurance. So go ahead, soak up the summer sun, and proudly display the flawless bikini line you've worked so hard to attain. Here's to your adventures, your attractiveness, and your amazing self-assurance.

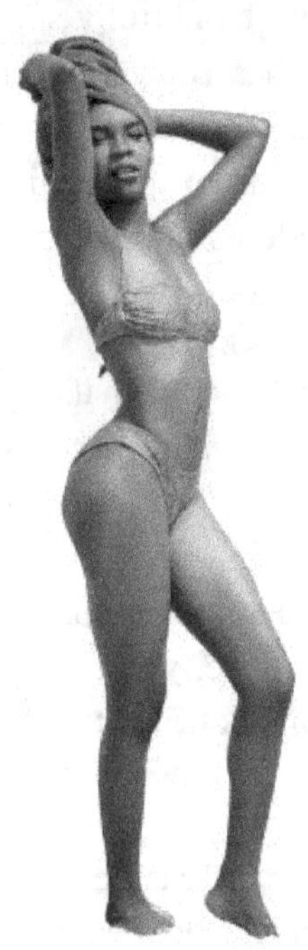